Table of Contents

The Relationship Between Nicotine and Anxiety: Connections, Feedback, Treatments, and More

The Relationship Between Nicotine and Anxiety: Connections, Feedback, Treatments, and More

1. Introduction to Nicotine and Anxiety

But there are other systems involved—some of which may be activated by nicotine itself. These include the body's primary stress response, the hypothalamic-pituitary-adrenal (HPA) axis, which is located in your brain. One of the primary hormones released by this system is cortisol. While cortisol regulates many systems in the body, researchers have found a few ways in which it might influence how much you smoke. Since smoking is something that also changes how your body responds to stress and anxiety, we were interested in looking for connections between smoking, anxiety, and the HPA axis. The work that you are about to read comes from a series of studies aimed at exploring these tangled relationships using both humans and animal models. To begin, I will discuss the relationship between smoking and anxiety, and pre-existing mental health conditions, before discussing the overlap and potential avenues of investigation of these relationships.

There is a strong and complex relationship between nicotine and anxiety. Research has shown this in a variety of ways. Anxiety affects smoking, but smoking can also affect anxiety, making it difficult to untangle the direction of these effects. Scientists have found a number of systems in the body that link nicotinic acetylcholine receptor (nAChR) signaling directly to anxiety. Some of these signals even play a part in controlling the HPA axis's response to stress.

2. Understanding Anxiety: Types, Symptoms, and Causes

Research has shown that there is a correlation between nicotine dependence and an increase in anxiety, thinking of anxiety as contributed to by two opposite things: attentional bias (where attention is drawn compulsively to the anxiety-causing stimulus) and cognitive avoidance. Researchers also believe that nicotine in itself works in a few different ways to induce a state of anxiety. The first way is through nicotine withdrawal, in which abstaining from smoking during the daily cycle of nicotine causes a biochemical craving which in turn disrupts mood. The second way that nicotine can induce anxiety is through the neurobiological response to smoking; even before smoking is taken up as a habit, the very first time can induce a relaxation effect which makes the user feel less anxious. This counterintuitive result means that once someone is addicted to nicotine, the pathways which reward a relaxing response become less efficient and thus anxiety is worsened through tobacco use. The causes and feedback of these causes are illustrated in figure 1.

Anxiety is something that many people suffer from in one way or another, but it can be a difficult term to define precisely. There are various types of anxiety disorders (ADs), including panic disorders, generalized anxiety disorders, post-traumatic stress disorders, and social phobias. Even with this wide spectrum, symptoms of an AD can include physical anxiety (such as shallow breathing and an increased heart rate), cognitive anxiety (such as difficulties concentrating), and behavioral anxiety (such as avoiding things that provoke fear). Additionally, the root of these symptoms varies from person to person but can include genetics, brain chemistry, life events, and personality. Furthermore, researchers have argued that these various components of anxiety often play off of each other and form something of a feedback loop.

3. The Science of Nicotine: Effects on the Body and Brain

The brain and body, once continuously exposed to nicotine, change. These changes can become ingrained in memory, in the affective quality of sensations and perceptions, and even in declarative or conscious cognition, in ways that make breaking the addiction extraordinarily difficult. Characterizing the roles of the pharmacologic effects of nicotine from the affective behavioral effects of smoking, and from the expectancy effects attendant to abstinence, is extremely difficult. Meditating on what aspects of the subject might be related to anxiety is the goal of this chapter. The reversal of these changes may require treatment with agents that either oppose these changes or assist in their repair and reversal.

Nicotine also has actions in inhibitory neurons of the brain by augmenting the release of GABA and decreasing the release of the inhibitory amino acid glycine in response. The modulatory actions of nicotine on local neurotransmitter release do not stop there. They extend to virtually all locations where nicotinic cholinergic receptors are found, including the ultimate processing machine of nature, the cerebral cortex, where mood, attention, and perception are ultimately created.

Once absorbed, nicotine activates nicotinic cholinergic receptors located on autonomic nerve endings and muscle fibers. Activation of these receptors releases multiple neurotransmitters locally, including acetylcholine, norepinephrine, dopamine, and glutamate, which produce various changes in glandular secretion, inflammation, and smooth muscle tone.

The wide currency of tobacco smoking reflects the fact that nicotine, the drug that makes cigarettes appealing, has demonstrated actions that affect every part of the body deeply implicated in maintaining health. These processes, once disturbed, are subjected to homeostatic negatives that restore normal activity through the application of allostatic principles. An examination of these actions reveals their effects on the body and brain.

4. Anxiety Disorders and Their Impact on Mental Health

At an individual level, these conditions can lead to significant personal suffering and functional impairment across multiple domains including health, social function, and emotional regulation. They are associated with increased odds of unhealthy behaviors, the use of psychoactive substances, interpersonal conflict, homelessness, unemployment, and increased risk of suicidal thoughts, attempts, and death. The links between nicotine use and smoking specifically to depression are well established, with increased prevalence and symptom severity in the former group outlined in detail. By contrast, evidence is more conflicting for anxiety disorders, and there appears to be something unique to panic disorder that distinguishes it from the wider group of anxiety disorders. Nonetheless, some research has hinted that these disorders may, in fact, initiate mood disturbances.

Anxiety disorders include panic disorder, social anxiety disorder, specific phobias, and generalized anxiety disorder, among others. With an estimated 33.7% of the global population affected by some form or another of anxiety in their lifetime, they have a significant impact on public health. Anxiety and anxiety disorders are often comorbid with other psychiatric disorders. For example, between 48-63% of individuals meeting the diagnostic criteria for depression at one point in time are estimated to also have an active anxiety disorder. Collectively, anxiety and anxiety disorders are the sixth leading determinant of years lived with disability.

5. Nicotine Use and Prevalence: Statistics and Trends

Some have suggested that while smoking may decrease, there will be a trend to increasing alternative forms of nicotine delivery, such as electronic cigarettes, although populations using complementary practices of smoking and non-smoking for nicotine are difficult to predict. Over the long term, rates of smoking in many Western countries are decreasing. For example, nearly 60% of men in developed countries smoked in the 1970s, but this figure had dropped to about 30% by the 1990s. Rates among U.S. adults have also dropped substantially since the 1960s, with only 17% of adults describing themselves as current smokers in 2011, as compared to 42% in 1965. In contrast, rates for women in developing countries and young people of both sexes in some countries have been, or continue to be, increasing. Overall, there are more deaths every year from smoking than a combination of deaths caused by AIDS, illegal drugs, alcohol, road accidents, suicide, and homicides in any given year.

The use of nicotine and products containing this highly addictive substance is widespread. This comprehensive overview will demystify nicotine use, and a number of additional reviews that are also in this journal offer detailed discussions of the many health effects of nicotine and how nicotine interacts with the brain and nervous system. Although we can look at different definitions of nicotine use and dependence, one approach puts the USA average at 28% of people using nicotine, and in some age groups as many as 50% using or having used with upcoming trends to reduce use of nicotine.

6. Biological Mechanisms of Nicotine and Anxiety Interactions

Nicotine's primary mechanism of action in the brain is through the nicotinic cholinergic receptors. Both fibers that use acetylcholine and norepinephrine are integral to the function of the LC and are key components of both the brain's arousal and central stress response systems. There is then a direct link in the brain between the brainstem arousal mechanism, the locus coeruleus (LC), the brain's key stress system, and the primary target of nicotine.

This entry will examine in fuller detail the points in the previous entry, such as how nicotine and nicotine withdrawal can influence mental states and how anxiety could increase the drive to seek nicotine. Adding to this, the current entry will examine potential interventions and how they work from a biological perspective. This entry will close with suggestions for the practitioner who has a client currently having problems with cigarette smoking or nicotine as it is used with vaping.

The effect that nicotine and anxiety have on each other makes some sense: because people report that they often smoke for stress relief, and because people who quit nicotine can report both anxiety and heightened stress, it would make sense if nicotine has the ability to mitigate anxiety and anxiety could increase the drive to use nicotine. Behaviourally and mentally this makes sense, but understanding the specific biological processes that control and maintain this relationship can help provide a deeper understanding of the nature of the relationship, and therefore provide a deeper understanding of potential interventions.

7. Psychological Factors in Nicotine and Anxiety Relationships

Interested readers may find similar mechanistic work and review articles in our original research and definitions of key terms. Such psychological and mechanistic data support construing nicotine as anxiolytic in nature, as nicotine reverses abstinence-evoked deficits in threat responding in paradigms that do not involve evaluation of direct associations between nicotine and negative affective states. These findings collectively converge on the suggestion that nicotine decreases negative affective states, particularly those inherently tied to the development and experience of anxiety, without implying a direct relationship between the two.

Psychological factors of the relationship between nicotine and anxiety. Further evidence exists for psychological factors contributing to the relationships between anxiety and nicotine. Research on panic psychopathology demonstrates that certain relationships in anxiety and nicotine are present in those who have panic disorders, but not in those with non-anxious psychiatric illness. In panic disorder, changes in withdrawal-related states, such as smoking urges and withdrawal symptoms, are associated with changes in state anxiety. This indicates that the relationship between nicotine use and anxiety levels is dynamic and can have a feedback effect. Such relationships are shown with the clearing of bolus cigarette nicotine and indiscriminate comedication (i.e., reliance on other anxiolytics) in panic disorder patients.

8. Behavioral Patterns and Coping Mechanisms in Nicotine Use for Anxiety

A very different explanation is important to also consider. Namely, when individuals feel stuck or believe that they cannot deal with their overall environment and that physical responses are intolerable, such as labile emotion, they often quit trying to reason with themselves and turn to the solace of anxiety medications and alcohol in an effort to self-medicate. The compulsive self-medication with drinks like alcohol may then exacerbate the physical ill-being of the individual including anxiety leading a negative feedback loop directly across time. The functioning of these neuroanatomical consequences is still unclear. However, recent data have suggested a positive correlation between the amygdala and anxiety that was directly related to the exacerbation of alcohol abuse.

Much has been written about how nicotine may treat anxiety, and various anatomical connections have been suggested. Cerebral data from positron emission tomography (PET) imaging, which observed regional cerebral blood metabolism in response to nicotine administration in anxiety disordered patients, have suggested a significant negative correlation in the amygdala. However, few have discussed the behavioral patterns and coping mechanisms that individuals diagnosed with anxiety disorders could develop and make automatic to cope with their fears. This relates to animal studies that often exist outside of the realm of nicotine showing that similar conditioning can occur with other drugs.

9. Dual Diagnosis: Nicotine Dependence and Anxiety Disorders

10. Epidemiological Studies on Nicotine and Anxiety Comorbidity

Many epidemiological studies examining the possible association between tobacco use and anxiety disorders were recently published. They have reached differing conclusions, the factors responsible for this heterogeneity being of different sorts, relating in general to sample selection, study design, study setting, and type of disorder. However, in the particular case of the association between substance misuse – in the majority of instances, the use of tobacco – and anxiety disorders, only a single literature review or meta-analysis was found among the consulted works, dealing with the relationship between panic disorder and the presence of nicotine addiction. Since the time of depositing this report, additional meta-analyses on the subject have been published. In point of fact, it is appropriate, in order to produce more general pictures, to distinguish between papers and reports classified as a function of the measure employed for anxiety. A range of indices and units of measure are employed in these works to evaluate anxiety symptoms or the presence of anxiety disorders. Generally speaking, these are related to the number of physical occurrences, or panic attacks, the presence of anxiety symptoms or of panic disorder as defined by DSM criteria. It may be useful to enumerate the different units in this connection: the prevalence of smoking in subjects affected or not by a depressive comorbidity, the odds ratio (OR) or risk of smoking, the presence of abuse and/or addiction substances, the consumption of tobacco or nicotine, suicide tobacco, and the prevalence of alcohol in populations having experienced anxiety disorder.

Summary: This chapter provides a global view of the comorbidity of nicotine use and psychiatric disorders in the general population, based on data from epidemiological surveys. The literature to which we have access is not unanimous regarding the comorbidity between nicotine use and anxiety disorders. The marked methodological differences of the studies considered prevent one from drawing general conclusions regarding comorbidity, particularly at the diagnostic level. It can only be affirmed that the consumption of tobacco in individuals suffering from anxiety is more frequent than in the general population, but the size of the effect varies greatly according to the nature of the studies considered. What is more, the results would vary depending on whether matched population controls or systematically recruited subjects are studied. New works, sufficient for exploring the relationship between panic disorder and tobacco use, will be needed to confirm these contentions. It is, in effect, necessary to bear in mind that certain authors have described comorbidity as vastly greater than the risk due to a common etiological or genetic factor.

11. Neurotransmitter Systems Involved in Nicotine and Anxiety

To begin to understand the relationship between nicotine and anxiety, we can look at the underlying neurotransmitter systems. This activity mainly regulates the major brain reward pathway and consists of the following: dopaminergic cell bodies in the VTA project to the NAc, with glutamatergic neurons from the prefrontal cortex facilitating this activity and GABA neurons from the NAc regulating the excitatory input from the VTA. Multiple neurotransmitter systems are involved in the relationship between nicotine and anxiety. The neurotransmitter systems influence the neuromodulatory effect of anxiety and their relationship with nicotine is discussed briefly below. Noradrenaline: The noradrenergic system is activated in response to excitement, its dysfunction results in depression and anxiety, and the noradrenergic stress system has been linked to panic disorders and PTSD.

Anxiety and nicotine use occur regularly and are continually related to one another. While attention has now been established at an increased risk of initiation of smoking and development of nicotine dependence in those with anxiety, there may also be a potential feedback loop where anxiety and the negative affect experienced during periods of withdrawal may be increased or prolonged via the effect of nicotine on mood correction. Tackling the relationship between nicotine intake and anxiety, therefore, offers insights into how these processes may either be nudged via treatment or buffer the detrimental effects of nicotine intake in clinical populations.

12. Genetic and Environmental Influences on Nicotine-Anxiety Connections

Building a multifaceted view of nicotine-anxiety connections is important in part because anxiety can prevent an individual from even starting to use various substances and substances especially prone to misuse, like nicotine. Other very early exposure opportunities frequently occur through environmental variables, perhaps most notably parental substance use that may be combined with an increased likelihood of antisocial behavior to use either just one of these as a delinquent coping method or combine both. Given that twin results suggest unique genetic contributions to the relationship between parenting stress and smoking, research might also distinguish between these persistent influences.

What causes some people to smoke when they are anxious, while others avoid smoking and turn to food for comfort when they are emotionally distressed? Importantly, the potential anxiety-reducing effects of nicotine may quickly translate into continued smoking and nicotine dependence. Understanding individual differences in underlying mechanisms that contribute to nicotine-anxiety connections may reveal who is at risk for perpetuated nicotine use, higher anxiety, or even the co-occurrence of an anxiety disorder. Genetic influences help determine our nicotine and anxiety relations, with environmental influences such as stress also adding complexity to these interconnections. At their intersection, anxiety is associated with changes in the "smoking/gene" interaction, which may cascade to PE in at least tobacco use.

13. Neuroimaging Research on Nicotine and Anxiety Responses

There is good reason to think that the comorbid depressive symptoms of that subgroup of clients are important to the anxiety responses reported by Najt and coworkers and the other three independent laboratories. Research with depressive and comorbid anxious-depressed participants conducted by Evatt and coworkers and reviewed and discussed earlier in this article, resembles at least some of the studies by Najt and coworkers. This research has suggested that somatic symptoms of anxiety predispose to anxiogenic nicotine-responses in depressed and anxious clients. Alteration of self-administered nicotine dose has been explored in only one positron emission tomography study of internet-based self-promises of double smokers.

The past decade has seen a rapid and substantial advance in neuroimaging research on the effects of nicotine or smoking on anxiety responses or states in healthy nonsmokers with varying degrees of symptoms of anxiety. The reviewed experiments report that nicotine and smoking produce significant anxiolysis or significant anxiogenesis in varying subgroups of anxious nonsmokers, depending on context. They include expectancy, intensity of threat, context of exposure to threat, and comorbid depressive symptoms. Future research will likely focus on individual difference variables related to this variation. The fact that independent laboratories have now reported increased symptoms of anxiety following nicotine in four subgroups of anxious clients brings an important caution to a nearly century-old axiom.

14. Clinical Presentation and Diagnostic Criteria for Nicotine-Induced Anxiety

Nicotine dependence disorder and nicotine withdrawal, with their clinical features of anxiety, are well delineated in the DSM-IV. Nicotine withdrawal has symptom criteria noted above, including usually depressed or irritable mood. The irritable mood in the setting of nicotine withdrawal that is not better accounted for by a depressive disorder can be alternatively presented as anxiety. Although it is outlined in the DSM-IV under differing diagnostic classes, the anxiety of nicotine withdrawal is generally part of the same clinical syndrome as nicotine dependence disorder. It is difficult to separate symptoms of nicotine withdrawal arising from the syndrome versus the actions of nicotine itself. Variables useful in the separation involve the intensity of withdrawal and its time of onset and depth. Generally, if the diagnosis of nicotine-induced anxiety can be made, the withdrawal criteria are likely met, and these symptoms will usually coexist in the same individual, making their separation an academic endeavor. It is important to note that in the current diagnostic criteria for nicotine dependence or nicotine withdrawal, there is no provision for the specification of an individual's leading symptom, as is generally considered useful for the clinical assessment and treatment of psychiatric disorders.

Diagnostic Criteria

The onset and duration of both acute and chronic nicotine use and abstinence have been discussed in preceding sections of this chapter. The onset of anxiety due to nicotine toxicity can present initially with any clinical effect but is often associated with immediate excessive intake of a nicotine product. The duration of nicotine-induced anxiety following a toxic ingestion is generally limited to less than 24 hours. The duration of anxiety following abrupt withdrawal is related to the intensity of nicotine intake, duration of abuse, and baseline anxiety in the individual. In general, the duration of this state of withdrawal is likely to be more severe or prolonged in the absence of other intoxicants, withdrawal states, or psychiatric illnesses.

Onset and duration

Clinical Presentation

15. Pharmacological Treatments for Nicotine Dependence and Comorbid Anxiety

Nowadays, nicotine dependence and anxiety disorders are progressively becoming the foci of increased interest. Smokers most of the time want to put an end to smoking. They may have started smoking in their adolescence. Nicotine dependence always coexists with other mental disorders, particularly anxiety disorders. Smoking initiation and abuse beginning in early adolescence may continue into adulthood. Addressing nicotine dependence in those individuals struggling with anxiety disorders is essential, which can be accomplished by thorough medical and pharmaceutical interventions. A number of substances have been shown to discourage smoking and reduce nicotine dependence. However, they may also be beneficial for other mental disorders, such as anxiety disorders. For evidence corroborating this, the findings discovered in existing reviews and meta-analyses, randomized controlled trials, guidelines, and scientific statements are considered helpful. The comorbidity of nicotine dependence and anxiety disorder through some pharmacological approaches is summarized in this article. The evidence was searched for clinical trials that used measures of tobacco use, such as smoking, nicotine levels, craving, quitting rates, and nicotine withdrawal symptoms, in randomized, double-blind, placebo-controlled study designs. The goal of this article is to examine the boundary of the pharmacological treatment of nicotine dependence and the comorbid anxiety disorder.

As it can be deduced from clinical findings, most smokers want to quit, and they begin to smoke in early adolescence. The issues related to nicotine dependence are of special interest to clinicians, public health, and policymakers. Nicotine dependence may coexist alongside other mental disorders, especially anxiety disorders. Providing treatment seems to be the most effective and practical step toward preventing the burdens associated with the comorbidity of nicotine dependence and anxiety. This can only be achieved by knowing the pharmacological interventions that have been efficacious at managing both nicotine dependence and anxiety disorder through empirical findings. The purpose of the present study is to perform a review to this effect. We began this study by identifying reviews, meta-analyses, randomized controlled trials, guidelines, and scientific statements related to the treatment of nicotine dependence and anxiety disorders via some pharmacological agents. We then conducted a search for empirical articles that met our selection criteria. Our search unearthed evidence of the clinical impact of varenicline for the treatment of nicotine dependence and comorbid anxiety, including generalized anxiety disorder, social anxiety disorder, and post-traumatic stress disorder.

16. Behavioral Therapies and Cognitive Interventions for Nicotine and Anxiety

1.1 The Use of Behavioral and Cognitive Treatment for Anxiety and Nicotine Use Some of the categories discussed here may or may not be considered "cognitive" or "behavioral" by definition or previous traditions. This paper sought to identify treatment interventions based upon the primary mode of treatment, rather than the traditional definition of whether they are behavioral or cognitive. For example, mindfulness meditation may involve cognitive changes, but this technique is taught in a behavioral manner, thus is considered a 'behavioral' intervention in this paper. Similarly, manipulations to generic cognitive restructuring, such as reappraisal techniques and thought challenging exercises, would generally be considered cognitive interventions. However, they require direct action of the individual and are thus discussed about the self-administered "behavioral" aspect that is often part of the practice. Finally, some of these treatments are less cognitive or behavioral in nature, but have the potential to address underlying biobehavioral concerns that would address either, or both, nicotine use and anxiety. For this reason, they are lumped into a related, but distinct category of treatment.

The use of the terms 'behavioral therapy', 'cognitive-behavioral therapy', 'behavioral interventions', 'cognitive interventions', and 'cognitive techniques' reveals the breadth of non-pharmacological approaches used to address both nicotine use and anxiety. In this section, we will address existing treatment for reducing behavioral and cognitive symptoms of nicotine and anxiety-related symptoms, highlighting both parallel treatments of the concern and focusing on interventions specific to one of the disorders in order to focus on the behavioral and cognitive components of each therapy.

17. Mindfulness and Relaxation Techniques in Nicotine Cessation Programs

This section of the text begins by focusing attention on mindfulness and relaxation techniques as therapeutic tools that can help manage cravings and symptoms related to smoking cessation, and explains how these techniques are incorporated in interventions in treatment programs based on nicotine deprivation. In the middle, the chapter discusses the importance of moderate to significant smoking underestimation in terms of the effectiveness of mindfulness and relaxation techniques. The main ideas that inspired the theoretical development and the objectives of this editorial and guide surround the functions of rituals associated with smoking related to handling affect and emotion, showing that this can moderate the effectiveness of the therapeutic techniques by predicting the levels of anxiety in response to the presentation of a withdrawal stimulus associated with the outcomes of this anxiety.

As indicated in the previous sections, currently there is a trend to incorporate non-pharmacological techniques for different toxic habits and addictions, not only for nicotine, that has been detected in the research on anxiety. Although at the beginning of the century their presence was somewhat rare, in recent years, especially in the last decade, there have been several investigations that have incorporated these techniques in order to be able to treat associated symptomology. In the case of nicotine, these are some of the most used relaxation and mindfulness techniques.

18. Alternative Therapies for Managing Nicotine Withdrawal and Anxiety Symptoms

18.2. Medical Cannabis: THC is also implicated in its ability to amplify the transmission of dopamine in the brain. The dopamine neurotransmitter helps control the brain's reward and pleasure centers. The overstimulation of the endocannabinoid system, in the exact brain regions that manage the reward system, is found to reproduce resources throughout the drug addiction cycle. Currently, two cannabinoid drugs - dronabinol (Marinol®) and nabilone (Cesamet®) - have been approved by the US FDA and other jurisdictions. ADHD is a risk factor for cigarette smoking and smoking cessation failure, as delayed maturation of the prefrontal cortex impairs its ability to exert "top-down" executive inhibitory control over subcortical "bottom-up" drives of addiction. Withdrawal from smoking in some individuals may ameliorate symptoms, including better response to ADHD stimulants. Combined stimulant therapy for both ADHD and nicotine dependence should be helpful in cases of partial response to nicotine withdrawal, and/or the patients' motivation to quit smoking is seriously low. This medication could not only reduce the side effects of nicotine withdrawal but also help increase the compliance of ADHD patients who are in smoking cessation therapy.

18.1. Morinda citrifolia (Noni): Morinda citrifolia (noni) is an evergreen tree originating in Southeast Asia and usually found in Polynesia. It possesses a large set of properties, including antioxidant, anti-inflammatory, lipid-reducing, and hypnotic effects. The hyponeuroadaptogen effects of M. citrifolia possess the ability to calm the person and stimulate energy without being excitatory. M. citrifolia ethanolic leaf extract modulates left frontal alpha as well as beta oscillatory activity involved in the synergy of behavioral bluntness and attentive force. Compared to the placebo, hypersynchronous alpha is reduced in the M. citrifolia group. Because these drugs are already in use in many psychiatric disorders, noni herbs may need to be further evaluated in the future.

19. Nicotine Replacement Therapies: Efficacy and Considerations

The remainder of this section will thoroughly review each nicotine replacement formulation individually. We will review what data are available that support the formulation, and we will provide sample recommendations and an overview of the strengths of the therapy. We will also review a variety of reasons and considerations to have in mind when considering a cessation strategy, especially one that includes the use of nicotine replacement. Later in this chapter, we will provide detailed information about adverse events and tolerability that should be considered for each formulation, as well as information on indications for use as provided with the recent package inserts. However, the package inserts do tend to be generic, and several external bodies have published guidelines for use of competing formulations – our data will do the same for each individual formulation. In addition, the DATA 2000 waiver eliminates much of the previous concern about the effects and tolerability of nicotinic therapy for the treatment of nicotine dependence, allowing physicians to treat this therapy as OTC in a general practitioner's office.

For many people with nicotine dependence, one strategy for managing withdrawal symptoms is to adopt nicotine replacement, or the detaching of the pleasure response from the innate pain relief of nicotine. The concept of nicotine replacement has been coupled with the belief that these nicotinic practices are dopamine-inducing behaviors, which offer a short-lasting reward, attach to pain relief, and ultimately cause paradoxical anxiety and pain, leading to avoidance by reduction. While many have suggested that getting tobacco users to adopt these therapies will help the truly dependent smokers continue to enjoy their nicotine, the veracity of the practice is still up for debate. There are a variety of methods of nicotine replacement, including the patch, gum, inhaler, lozenge, nasal spray, and perhaps soon, vaccines that would allow the immune system to target nicotine for removal from one's body. This chapter attempts to present the data on nicotine replacement efficacy in an ordered and systematic way so that these practices can be thought about more rationally.

20. Impact of Nicotine Use on Anxiety Medications and Vice Versa

Looking from the other lens, the anxiety medications that an individual uses also impacts the likelihood that he or she will or will not use nicotine. This is demonstrated by an interrelationship study that showed previous nicotine use behaviors did not encourage future benzodiazepine use. Here's what I mean about nicotine use interfering with the effectiveness of anxiety meds: Researchers have shown that when people addicted to alcohol and other sedatives take benzodiazepines, they might be more likely to smoke. This is because benzodiazepines, including Valium and Xanax, have been found to work as GABA or gamma-aminobutyric acid, which reduces stress and anxiety by preventing neurons in the brain from becoming overactive and overwhelming. Even in adults with the mobile social anxiety associated with autism, the anti-anxiety effects of benzos can be significantly boosted if they are used in combination with cigarettes. On the other hand, for instance, when people quit smoking, sedative effects from benzos including Valium and Xanax are dramatically enhanced.

Just knowing that an individual who uses nicotine also uses an overweighted medication is a promising first step in identifying potential treatment targets and sharing therapy between these two behaviors. For example, why not present the treatment pathways for both behaviors at the same time? This is particularly important since nicotine use can reduce some of the anxiety-reducing effects of many anxiety medications, including antidepressants and benzodiazepines.

Topic: Looking at the relationship between anxiety medications and nicotine, a new study reveals that a huge 40% of smokers report using benzodiazepines just in the past year. On the flip side, individuals who use such meds have been found to be more likely to use nicotine as well. Based on their findings, researchers see a clear need for interventions that work to address both benzodiazepine use and nicotine use at the same time.

21. Public Health Policies and Interventions for Nicotine-Induced Anxiety

Public health has long recognized that a key to curbing the tobacco epidemic is creating smoke-free work and public spaces, says Anne Hartman, the director of tobacco control resources and initiatives for the American Lung Association. According to Hartman, another strike-off process to reduce anxiety upon quitting is having tobacco regulations that maintain restricted usage of nicotine, such as sending prescriptions and nicotine replacement therapy-free or discounted options to the intrusively poor or uninsured. Creating an environment with strict enforcement of tobacco regulations by officials and non-tobacco use by the public contributes to relinquishing some of the mindsets and facilitators that maintain such anxiety about quitting, she said, but you need to get through the door to done some day.

Smoking, similar to nicotine, is interrelated with anxiety. However, research about the connections between nicotine and anxiety remained sparse until the 1990s. reported that anxiety sensitivity was a consistent mediator for those with cigarette smoking to experience panic attacks and panic disorder. In 1999, stated that only a few studies had examined the relationship between nicotine and anxiety regarding panic disorder. Consequently, less is documented about public health policies, campaigns, and interventions to target or accommodate the nexus of nicotine and anxiety. Putting the spotlight on such viable interventions matters given the high rates of coexperienced anxiety and behavior of nicotine use and smoking cigarettes.

22. Educational Campaigns and Awareness Programs on Nicotine-Anxiety Links

There is a lack of dedicated initiatives aimed at increasing knowledge and consciousness of these things. Efforts would need to be granted support and funding to cover things such as content preparation, dissemination, and evaluation. At the same time, there also exists compelling evidence that community-based education programs can be helpful (and there are some available statistics and recommendations of good practices). That is partly the intent and scope of the present paper. It identifies the several knowledge-based experience of interested others and pulls on those to put forward several basic ideas on how we can raise awareness and facilitate community education regarding the connections between nicotine and anxiety. More descriptive guidance on how to conduct these awareness programs needs to be drawn and developed.

Researchers and experts can be quite removed from their communities, and information about the links between nicotine and anxiety isn't always the most accessible. Several research teams and experts have put substantial effort into developing educational campaigns and awareness programs to assist in disseminating information about the connections between nicotine and anxiety. These campaigns and programs all share a key commonality: they aim to elevate the general knowledge and awareness of the multitude of relationships between nicotine use and anxiety by educating, approaching, and engaging in activities where the research community, practitioners, and the general public have some level of interest, stakes, and consciousness about those relationships. The issues raised above, and more, have led to suggested recommendations for the development and launch of awareness programs based on relevant literature, knowledge, and resources.

23. Community Support and Resources for Individuals with Dual Nicotine and Anxiety Concerns

Search by location and issue to find therapists and psychiatrists willing to work with folks with anxiety and/or nicotine use, and also read and post local ads for "Support Groups." Let's face it; taking the steps to get away from the mind bend of nicotine is full of insane anxiety until the turmoil starts to ebb. Browse here for not just the AA groups, but also the anxiety groups. Often reading a bit about other people's experiences will help individuals in many ways. The app and website "Meetup" can be looked up as well; one of my best friends found a local "Vaping Recovery" group through this site, and it turned out to be an absolutely wonderful resource.

This is often a helpful place to check out before doing a larger internet search or diving into the deep world of psychology, drugs, and medical literature. NIDA tends to be and tries to stay up to date on current well-researched information about drugs of abuse, and often partners with public health institutions and private doctor's groups also provide sometimes very helpful, clearly written reports for the education of the general population.

One of the most beneficial facets of having a community, in person or online, is its ability to remind one that they are truly not alone. Struggling with both nicotine and the possibility of worsening anxiety because of that?

Understand that there are many other people contending with the same problems. They offer a perspective that is often difficult to grasp from such an inward position. Others, particularly in support groups, can also help a person brainstorm and think through their individual issues and strategies.

24. Ethical Considerations in Research on Nicotine and Anxiety Relationship

The existence of a reciprocal anxiety-smoking feedback loop is not entirely clear. But examining and finding a causal relationship between nicotine or smoking and anxiety is a fundamental area. Is it somehow ethical to put people at risk for gaining an anxiety disorder in order to learn more about gardening? In fact, studying the association between anxiety and nicotine can only and often unintentionally harm a smoker during his or her life.

It is clear that there are many ways in which anxious symptoms and smoking uninhibited are harmful to human health both physically and mentally (e.g., it is harmful for pregnant women's blood pressure to go up when they're anxious). Given the nature of the relationship between smoking and anxiety, it seems to be the right thing to do ethically to study this relationship (as we can help many people suffering from anxiety symptoms). The connections we have been examining can reveal to us the potential interference that may have made smokers more susceptible to stress and the deterioration of emotional resilience in the 21st century, as well as help us to more deeply understand the underlying neuropathology in smokers and the alterations that smoking may have made in the use of targeting drugs. But proceeding with full knowledge of the nature of the topic increases the responsibility an investigator would have not to expose their subjects to additional anxiety-related harm, and to avoid advertising that could potentially implicate additional stress or reinforce negative stereotyping to those smoking subjects struggling with anxious control. Continuing research may uncover a range of possible therapeutic targets and treatment modifiers for smokers, the existence of which human subjects may be interested in. However, due to the harm that could occur from nicotine and tobacco-based medication, and their potential for misuse, future investigation of these areas would require more stringent assumptions, careful consideration, and cautious consideration as to the beneficiaries.

25. Future Directions and Emerging Trends in Nicotine-Anxiety Research

There is also scope for the further development of qualitative research in this field. Given that GAD is a particularly common anxiety disorder and it has helped to elucidate core features of excessive anxiety which may relate to all types of anxiety among smokers, examining this state in further detail using mixed methodology, including laboratory work, will enhance our understanding of potential mechanisms and informative phenotypes. It is anticipated that there will also be increased academic and clinical focus on NRT treatment examining both efficacy and predictors of response among those with an anxiety disorder. Future research will also consider whether dual step-down models and combined treatments analogous to those for the treatment of comorbid mood disorders may be useful in the treatment of anxiety.

There are several future directions and emerging trends in the field of nicotine-anxiety relationship research. This includes the possibility that the presentation of anxiogenic states could be examined in the natural environment using ecological momentary assessment. Additionally, given that the preponderance of data have arisen from cross-sectional studies, the design and execution of prospective research studies is likely to be of increasing interest. Based on the improvements observed with some behavioral and psychological treatments for anxiety in smokers and within specialized services for anxiety, treatments and outcomes

in these groups might be evaluated, taking into account
potential moderators such as the type and severity of the
anxiety, as well as comorbid conditions.

26. Conclusion: Key Findings and Implications for Clinical Practice and Policy

Implications for policy The policy implications of this research are to increase both content and effectiveness of integrated treatments for tobacco use and other components of the syndrome(s) of emotional suffering. Policy changes favoring truly integrated care will lead to a major change in the thinking of tobacco control funding bodies as well as those of clinical mental health services, and smoking-related work should be seen as part of a long-term recovery plan for the mentally ill. In the USA (and perhaps elsewhere), such work is not traditionally considered 'health promotion'. Work that starts to close this gap is certainly on the near horizon in the nation's public mental health agencies, which provide services to a large cohort of people who have histories of high tobacco use as outpatients and many who smoke inpatient psychiatric hospitals. In these large treatment systems, labor, property, and insurance resources are available, and the matter of fashioning a wise and sustained use of them is a pressing one. More intimate and effective conversations among basic scientists interested in anxiety and nicotine, clinicians seeing a panoply of smokers, and smokers managing anxiety on a daily basis are timely and necessary.

Implications for clinical practice Although patients may experience some initial increase in anxiety when attempting to quit smoking, increased anxiety is less a hallmark of long-term abstinence than is often feared. Behavioral counseling and anxiolytic medications like SSRIs are important adjuncts to the nicotine agonist therapy. The clinician should make an extra effort to repeatedly emphasize the progressive reduction of anxiety in the long-term after smoking cessation. In anxious smokers with extant comorbid anxiety disorders, appropriate pharmacotherapy should be offered, and depression should be carefully treated.

Key findings The available literature suggests that there may indeed be a complex and potentially vicious feedback cycle between nicotine use and anxiety disorders. At the biological level, nicotinic mechanisms may exacerbate the stress response, whereas hypoactive dopaminergic and noradrenergic metabolisms may create a self-perpetuating cycle of anxiogenesis, nicotine use to decrease negative cognitive-affective states, and enhanced stress system reactivity after nicotine administration. The psycho-social vulnerability factors for both nicotine use and anxiety disorders appear predominantly similar, e.g., developmental stress/genetic influences and cocaine-use-related development of hyperdopaminergic anxiety. In clinical practice, taking into account the bidirectional effects of nicotine on anxiety may be helpful for developing more effective anxiety treatment strategies in anxious smokers.

27. References

Anda, R. F., Williamson, D. F., Escobedo, L. G., Mast, E. E., & Giovino, G. A. (1990). Depression and the dynamics of smoking. JAMA: Journal of the American Medical Association, 264, 1541-1545. Bierut, L.J. (2010) Convergence of genetic findings for nicotine dependence and smoking-related diseases with chromosome 15q24-25. Trends in Pharmacological Sciences, 31(1), 46-51. Caggiula, A.R., Donny, E.C., Palmatier, M.I., Liu, X., Chaudhri, N., & Sved, A.F. (2009). The role of nicotine in smoking: A dual-reinforcement model. In M. C. S. L. Bickel (Ed.). Aversive Interpersonal behaviors. The Guilford Press. March Gilbert, D.G., McClernon, F.J., Rabinovich, N.E., Dibb, W.D., Plath, L.C., Hiyane, S.D., et al. (2002). Mood disturbance fails to resolve across 31 days of cigarette abstinence in women. Journal of Consulting and Clinical Psychology, 70, 142-52. Parrott, A. C. (1992). The psychopharmacology of everyday life. British Journal of Social Psychology, 31(2), 145-164. Radzius, A., Gallo, J. J., Epstein, A. E., Eaton, W. W., & Bruce, M. L. (2003). Anxiety disorders and use of nicotine and other psychoactive drugs. Drug and Alcohol Dependence, 70, 61-68. Verplaetse, T.L., Weinberger, A.H., Smith, P.H., Cosgrove, K.P., Mineur, Y.S., Picciotto, M.R., Mazure, C.M., McKee, S.A. (2017). Targeting the dysregulated stress-responsive HPA axis with a dual NPY Y1/Y5 receptor antagonist may yield improved smoking cessation therapies. European Neuropsychopharmacology, 27(11), 1098-1109.

The Relationship Between Nicotine Products and Anxiety: Understanding the Short-Term Relief and Long-Term Consequences

1. Introduction to Nicotine Products and Anxiety

In this article, we explore the relationship between the use of nicotine products and anxiety. We first explain how nicotine products provide short-term relief from anxiety. We then look at the ways in which long-term nicotine use can result in higher levels of anxiety. Finally, we discuss ways to help break free from nicotine addiction.

Nicotine is a type of mind-altering product that can be found in a handful of products that are consumed for recreational purposes. It can change a person's thinking, make them feel happier or more relaxed, and it can be addictive. When it comes to nicotine products, many of them, including cigarettes and vape pens, claim to help reduce feelings of stress and anxiety which can be quite attractive to individuals with high levels of anxiety. The problem is that while these products may have an initial calming effect, they can actually end up increasing anxiety in the long run. Nicotine is a habit-forming stimulant and as a person's use of these products increases, their anxiety can also increase. This creates a cycle of use that can be very difficult to break.

2. The Short-Term Effects of Nicotine Products on Anxiety

Anxiolytic Derby Hypothesis. In short, it is those habits that precede nicotine administration that can have an anxiolytic impact upon people looking forward to those adverse experiences, not the nicotine itself. The quadratic relationship between premorbid anxiolytic smoking-induced relaxation (DKK13) and post-morbid state anxiety reduction score (A-AD, analogue of A-VAS-DK) was mediated by parallel arousal reduction. Identical high levels of arousal for individuals taking both high and low levels of on-arousal tobacco smoke preceded the highest ratings of relaxation-and-arousal combination, i.e. greater state mood relaxation. The anxiety-increasing tension reduction path predicts non-anxiolytic passive habituation to adverse anticipation (tethering).

Physiological Mechanisms. When put in terms of immediate satisfaction, few anxiolytic strategies have as quick and as long-lasting effects on acute anxiety as consuming nicotine. Smokers report that cigarettes provide instant relief from anxiety, reduce stress, and give pleasurable feelings. Also, smoking has these immediate anxiolytic effects even in non-anxious but negative affective states. Giving nicotine to non-smoking regular tea and coffee consumers reduces stress and enhances the relaxation associated with the morning ritual. All forms of nicotine (cigarettes, gum, inhaler, and nasal spray) reduce symptoms of dysphoria, depression, and nausea among people with schizophrenia. Also, nicotine tends to alleviate clinical anxiety disorders. The stress-buffering and pain-reducing effects of nicotine last for many hours on a single dose and occur instantly after each dose.

Physical anxiety is an all-over-the-body feeling of raised alertness to a threat that is either real or perceived. It's a combination of hormones and physiological reactivity to a concern. When anxiety comes down to worry, this feeling is decreased by nicotine intake, and so the very natural one will try to maintain the very low worry level to avoid the worry sensation. The body relies on the hormone process instead of bodily processes; the natural ones want to worry, but the hormones are not raised enough to worry. That is reduced first through the conscious act, so one will take a deep satisfying drag from a cigarette to remove a steady concern as they light it. The nicotine then engages the liver to supply the simple sugar found at the brain synapse that relieves concern, and from here opposes the improved time it would take the nicotine to pass into the bloodstream through the lungs.

However, caffeine and nicotine are two of the biggest contributors to this kind of feeling. When the hormonal adjustment of an individual alters with commercial products such as caffeine and nicotine of any form that are present in various products such as energy drinks, cigarettes, snuff, and smokeless tobacco, they have a direct effect on the regulation of anxiety in the brain. This physiological mechanism has both short and long-term effects on individuals over time who rely on nicotine. The physiological mechanism in which individuals feel less anxiety when using nicotine.

2.2. Psychological Impact

Nicotine, in the most immediate and direct way, helps modulate overwhelming states: alienation, overstimulation, impulse. In the moment of stressful disorientation, it will reproportion the self and the world in mutually reassuring dimensions, if only briefly. Withdrawal or abstinence leaves an individual highly irritated or unable to concentrate. Those who have documented high rates of comorbidity between various anxiety disorders or depression with substance abuse/dependence argue that underlying psychopathology leads individuals to use substances such as nicotine in order to self-medicate or alleviate their symptoms. They also cite studies showing that substance use disorders commonly precede the onset of specific anxiety disorders, and that daily users of nicotine are diagnosed with an anxiety disorder more frequently than non-users.

A previously unexamined angle concerning the relationship between nicotine products and stress is their immediate psychological impact. Calming oneself with a Nicorette (nicotine gum) or by smoking a cigarette is not just a sensual response. It is a psychological act, in the same category as a self-soothing technique. Nineteen of our participants mentioned being told to use deep breathing exercises when stressed, some in therapeutic settings. These clients are given the message, in effect, "don't smoke, do something else." Consequently, they see deep breathing as "replacing" the cigarette or the Nicorette. Participants confirmed that clients who smoke or use Nicorette generally do not like deep breathing, and even consider it to be ineffective. Bottled scents or oils - "aromas" - can be another self-soothing technique; and this comparison is flattening the essential pace of all relationships.

3. The Development of Dependence on Nicotine Products

There is a wide variety of etiological factors that contribute to developing a product use habit including the expectancies users have of a product, and in the anxiety-management part of the model, as they are also thinking of learned habit behaviors within other models. When expectancies are involved in the process of changing how one feels and when learned habits are complete, they can create situations where individuals are tricked into feeling positive or stress-free emotions as they engage in specific behaviors. For many, using a mode at currently low levels - such as vaping - is a calculated enjoyment seen as a breather or break, which they actively seek through cues as we saw in the study. In other individuals, with vastly different relationships with nicotine products, such as someone with high susceptibility to developing a smoking habit, reactivity to stress increases use/escalates behavioral habits between cue and use. The development of these habit behaviors increases use as the novelty of the other reactivity decreases.

There are several factors involved in the development of not just a dependence on nicotine products in general, but specifically the onset of dependence on nicotine products as a mode of anxiety relief. Part of the development of this dependence lies, in part, in the effectiveness of nicotine products in relation to their anxiolytic effects. Nicotine oversees the release of less stimulating neurotransmitters and causes the increase of calming neurotransmitters. This creates the illusion of stress relief within an individual experiencing such relief. This can make a previously "low road" emotion (stress) that one experiences in stages of a panic disorder, for example, into something that they tolerate more and more and look for in their life and in product use. On the habit formation side, tough days raise cue-driven links to nicotine treatment, triggering cravings and using behaviors.

3.1. Neurobiological Factors

A dependence on nicotine products is accompanied by structural alterations in the brain, as well as in the levels of chemicals within the body which control attention, stress, and pleasure. Once a person becomes dependent on nicotine, any downregulation of dopamine as a consequence of stress (i.e., at a physiological level) is perceived far more than in those without a nicotine dependence, which can precipitate feelings of irritability and stress, as mentioned above. This relationship between the reduced effect of nicotine upon dopamine release results in the physical necessity for nicotine 'top-ups' to manage low mood and irritability, creating a vicious circle. At the behavioural level, each time someone with a nicotine dependence smokes, they offer themselves temporary relief from stress or negative mood; ergo, they find an increase in gratification and belief that hardships are more manageable. When smokers are anxious, a cigarette can offer temporary relief; their body chemistry has been modified, and whilst nicotine can provoke anxiety, not smoking can create a temporary relief from the increased effects of stress seen as a consequence upon the body chemistry. Withdrawal symptoms are due in part to build-up of the increased activity of the nerves and nervous system that occurs as a consequence of the downregulation of the fight-or-flight response. If a smoker quits a product containing nicotine, symptoms linked with nervous system over-activity can result (see anxiety and panic symptoms). The body's carbon monoxide level also reduces when the smoker stops. Carbon monoxide attaches to red blood cells that normally carry oxygen. As such, minimal oxygen intake is seen. This means that vital organs are not receiving enough energy despite burning glucose. Blood glucose is taken from storage and usually reduces as a result. Brain cells need glucose to function optimally.

3.2. Psychological Factors

However, psychology also involves desire as a motivation. "Craving," or the psychological urge to smoke, is a counterpart to the person's preference for smoking, especially when abstinent, when the horizons leading to smoking seem so open. Those with high impulse buying preferences may see smoking as one of many similar high-risk activities to also be indulged. The relief from withdrawal symptoms would accompany this craving and may also act as a reinforcer, not just because relief removes unpleasantness, but because relief becomes pleasurable again to the addict's senses and self-sense. The non-smoker feels threatened and may engage in crepitation (nostril opening) as a part of an infantile or germ-phobic dealing with anxiety. The smoker, initially or in times of stress, will either increase smoking, continue smoking, or, as a genetic condition of non-dependent type, predictably reduce use. Social comfort data on age of first smoking, for example, suggests that cigarettes can be smoked at the youngest age, followed by using a pipe, then tobacco chewing, and finally cigars. In Tanzania, 30% of the adults of the Masai tribe chew only tobacco, with a mean intake of 400g/week.

Psychological factors: Experimentation with tobacco use for many new users is often based on curiosity or may be incidental to exposure or to relieve external or psychic stress, where smoking may produce a sense of increased alertness and decreased stress. For some adolescents, smoking signifies independence, while conditions that increase anxiety or social awkwardness may initially increase smoking as a part of association and rebellion. On the positive side, when smoking is motivated by friendliness and with no indicators of egotism or smoking as an invitation to social situations, smoking is less likely to be a way to cope with social anxiety. As these studies suggest, psychological explanations of the continuation of drug use tend to involve a preference for independent and social interaction. When this social acceptance and tolerance of drug use is absent, so too are the concepts that describe this prohibition. Psychology in the use of tobacco nicotine, however, goes beyond choosing based not on tolerance and nicotine's reward in the brain.

4. The Cycle of Anxiety and Nicotine Dependence

One is easy to see and understand. As regular users of nicotine products feel the physical consequences of going without for even just a few hours, their chemical dependence is translated into conscious, negative mood states. In effect, every day tens of thousands of people going through nicotine withdrawal effectively feel "anxiety-ridden" as a result. Nicotine is also observed to increase the activity of certain neurotransmitters that are also released during exercise in emotionally uplifting ways. For these and other reasons, smoking has an immediate and reinforcing impact on neurotransmitters such as norepinephrine, dopamine, and serotonin. Furthermore, regular use of nicotine products can also blunt the receptors for corticotropin and other stress-related hormones, leading these and other users to feel more "baseline" happiness. It's a pessimistic and seductive siren song. It offers ease of mind and relief in the short term before requiring increased dependence for the same effect and lowering overall quality of life in the long term.

Certainly, in the beginning, nicotine products, be they cigarettes or vape products, seem to provide relief to the troubles of anxiety. Many of us report anxiety relief and improved mood upon using tobacco products, a phenomenon which has been demonstrated and researched over and over again. However, things are not always so simple. There is a very complicated and long-lasting interplay between anxiety and tobacco use, with each of them resulting from and carefully reinforcing the other.

5. Strategies for Quitting Nicotine Products

Nicotine dependence is 70% heritable, making a genetic contribution to the motivation for stopping nearly certain. Smoking cessation clinicians speak of pharmacogenomics, as it pertains to the likelihood of someone representing a "good" responder or a "slow" responder to NRT, based upon which of two amino acids they carry at chromosome 15, across the nicotinic receptors located cornerstone in the level of brain in addiction development and maintenance. Nonspecific effects of medications (non-selective MAO inhibitors, bupropion and nortriptyline) may replicate the higher quit rates possible with these medications. There are strengths and power in doing so. Intervention options for the dissemination of effective treatments encompass pharmacological, individual and group counseling. There were modest to no differences in effectiveness in quitting between group and individual counseling delivery through the Quitlines. Population-based delivery of quitline services save years of life, are cost effective.

A multitude of behavioral therapy programs have been developed for tackling tobacco/nicotine dependence. These typically address both the positive reinforcing properties of the drug, as well as the negative reinforcing properties of withdrawal. Additionally, a substantial research base has been built for the use of various pharmacological treatments including: NRT, bupropion, varenicline, and the recently approved levetiracetam. The positive effects of each of these drugs can be ascribed to actions that they have at the level of the nicotinic cholinergic receptors, suggesting that the target of medication development continues to be the nicotine molecule.

5.1. Behavioral Interventions

Behavioral interventions or strategies with or without e-cigarette cessation medication can be adopted. The components included in behavioral strategies can be tailored according to user preference, and relevant information can be shared according to current requirements. The organization's healthcare providers can be trained to assist in helping others quit. Simple cessation techniques are, however, implemented for critical users to prevent all types of tobacco while receiving hospital care. Individuals interested in quitting with a professional expert can be invested in more time. Priorities for quitting substance use can be recommended according to the patients' capacities and the potential for developing tobacco-related diseases and conditions resulting from sudden death. Behavioral strategies often include techniques such as setting target dates for quitting, making strategies, and drawing on the capability of recovery and medication. Relapses are generally quick and relaxed with an emphasis on positive and informative ways to stay tobacco-free.

In this context, behavioral interventions are found to be appropriate among vaping populations, especially among short-term e-cigarette quitters or those interested in quitting e-cigarettes. Government-approved behavioral therapy is also successful. Meanwhile, studies also found that psycho-educational intervention in addition to nicotinic replacement did not reduce Singaporean e-cigarette users' nicotine dependence, although it was effective in helping them to quit e-cigarettes.

Overall, smoking cessation or quitting is considered as the only way to escape from the complications. Yet, only 40%-70% find behavioral interventions exceptionally difficult for the majority of Indian individuals as the first step to quit. However, a lower success rate was noted among individuals with a nicotine dependence ranging from 13% to 2.5%.

5.2. Pharmacological Treatments

NRTs such as nicotine patches, gum, and lozenges address the craving for nicotine, although most people do not succeed in quitting smoking long term. Research on the inability of NRTs to help people quit successfully has led scientists to hypothesize that other factors such as sensory contributions to the habit of smoking play a role in the continued use of cigarettes as well as e-cigarettes, heated tobacco devices, and snus. Research studies with medications to treat both psychological and nicotine cravings and habits have been encouraging. However, some other studies suggest caution should be employed when using a combination of different medications when stopping nicotine products, to avoid particles combining that could, for example, increase seizure risk. More research is needed before some of these combinations can be recommended to the public. Medical approaches to assist weaning and reducing consumption neglected the psychological habit and received little interest after positive results had been published. Management of anxiety associated with nicotine cessation uses psychological approaches.

A number of pharmacological treatments are now available to assist individuals to manage or overcome their dependence on different nicotine products such as cigarettes, liquids for electronic cigarettes, and loose snus. In recent years, topiramate, baclofen, and varenicline have been studied as agents to treat the physical dependence rather than the psychological habit of smoking. When used as standalone treatments or in combination with other approaches, varenicline (Chantix, Champix) and bupropion (Zyban) have each been shown helpful in discontinuing cigarettes and e-cigarettes in clinical trials.

Subsection 5.2. Pharmacological Treatments

6. The Importance of Support Networks

Consider who you trust and with whom you would be willing to share your experience with using e-cigarettes or quitting using nicotine products. Support from friends and family can range from practical or emotional support, such as going for walks, using face masks, or watching movies for self-care. Friends and family can also serve as an important distraction or coaches by teaching and supporting positive coping strategies. Some individuals have links to community or nationwide organizations that provide a network of coaches who also support people as they learn to better manage their mood without nicotine. These links are to websites that identify a program or group that has gathered to share experiences and strategies on how to quit without using nicotine. Talking with others who have been successful can provide insight into how to join groups. It can be helpful, and support may be offered and received over the phone, in person, or via chat website application.

Living without nicotine is possible. This guide explains the short-term and long-term changes that e-cigarettes, tobacco, and nicotine products have in relation to anxiety levels. If you currently struggle with anxiety, depression, or substance use, it is important to seek the support of a mental health, substance use, or social worker professional. A physician can help you explore medication and methods to overcome anxiety that do not include e-cigarettes, vape, or tobacco. It is important to tell a doctor that you want to use e-cigarettes to help with anxiety, depression, or quitting tobacco. A doctor should be aware of the risks and help the individual evaluate the long-term outcomes.

7. Long-Term Benefits of Quitting Nicotine Products

In addition to the relaxation stemming from not being dependent on a given substance, there are numerous physical and mental benefits of refraining from the use of nicotine. These include, but are not limited to, a decreased overall risk of mortality and severe health problems, stronger immunity, improved sense of taste and smell, reduced likelihood of cardiac-related medical issues, healthier lungs, greater likelihood of becoming pregnant, regained ability to exercise and be active, the return of healthy, glowing skin, fresh breath, and yellowing teeth.

Despite the belief that smoking provides those with anxiety a form of relief, Leventhal assures that this is not actually the case. In fact, once individuals are about fifteen years removed from smoking their last cigarette, this relief from anxiety that nicotine had once provided has dissipated, making anxiety worse for the long-term. "For the first one to three years, people who do quit may feel worse. But afterwards, they will feel a lot better than they would have if they had continued to smoke. These findings should reassure people with high anxiety that quitting will be currently beneficial."

A study published in Scientific Reports by Professor Adam Leventhal of the Keck School of Medicine of the University of Southern California specifically targeted smokers with anxiety in order to determine how they differ from other smokers. The results from the study indicated that smokers with a high level of anxiety relative to non-anxious smokers were significantly more dependent upon nicotine and had more trouble quitting due to stronger withdrawal symptoms.

These withdrawal symptoms can be addressed in a number of different ways, including alternative forms of nicotine ingestion, certain medications, additional support from mental health professionals, or a combination of any of these three strategies. It is often worth mentioning the long-term good that can come as a result of quitting nicotine, as it could provide some reassurance and incentive to those struggling with the idea of giving up the products that have offered them relief for so long.

8. Conclusion and Future Directions

Given the vast body of evidence from both laboratory and clinical research implicating nicotine in the direct cause of anxiety and panic in humans, it is surprising that it is not mentioned in the DSM-V as a possible pharmacological cause of panic disorder. This, combined with the observation that many individuals with anxiety disorders use nicotine products to self-medicate anxiety, suggests that much more research is needed to understand the interactions between nicotine and mood states and disorders at both neurobiological and cognitive levels of analysis. The elimination of these unknowns will provide medical and psychological professionals the knowledge needed to develop and implement the most effective and individually tailored prevention, intervention, and treatments. This could also prevent a substantial portion of the population from beginning to use or continuing to use a product that contributes to the major causes of death and disability in individuals with these disorders.

Given the well-established connection between nicotine products, anxiety, and mood disorders, it is unsurprising that many individuals use nicotine products to attempt to self-medicate negative emotions. The majority of both experimental and survey-based studies on the relationship between nicotine products and anxiety support the hypothesis that nicotine temporarily relieves anxiety. However, these short-term effects can have longer-term consequences, such as increasing negative affect and dependence on nicotine products. Pharmacological research has uncovered complex relations between nicotine and anxiety at both biological and cognitive levels. However, no evidence supports a consistent or stable anxiolytic effect of nicotine, or PCCs as a whole, in humans.

www.ingramcontent.com/pod-product-compliance
Lightning Source LLC
Chambersburg PA
CBHW061005260726
48661CB00005B/2061